Chronic kidney disease (CKD) is a worldwide health condition that has no age barrier. In North America, over 26 million people are affected with CKD and thousands use dialysis as a way to prolong life.

The book begins with an overview of the kidneys. It explains dialysis—what it is, how it works, what to expect, and the different types available. It offers tips on, cleaning solutions, support systems, renal diet, sex, cramping, exercise, travel, and other feel-good therapies.

A Helping Hand On Dialysis offers help to patients and their families who are undergoing kidney dialysis. Written by a dialysis patient who draws on her 11 years experiences, happily managing the treatment.

Alexander shows how you can adapt to the lifestyle changes and continue to enjoy this big beautiful world while maintaining a healthy lifestyle. She offers solutions to handle the hardship, fears, and anxiety associated with dialysis.

An invaluable resource for coping both physically and emotionally with a chronic condition from a patient point of view.

A must read. Get your copy.

A HELPING HAND ON DIALYSIS:

POWER TIPS TO ENHANCE THE DIALYSIS LIFE

CLAUDETTE ALEXANDER

A HELPING HAND ON DIALYSIS:
Power Tips To Enhance The Dialysis Life
By Claudette Alexander

Publisher: SABU PRESS
Toronto, Ontario, Canada
Email: calex999@sympatico.ca

Interior kidney illustrations: Terence Hyacinth
Cover Design: Rigers Popa

Library and Archives Canada Cataloguing
National Archives Authority of Saint Lucia
A Helping Hand On Dialysis: Power Tips To Enhance The Dialysis Life/
Claudette Alexander 1950
ISBN: 978-09936386-2-6 (Electronic version)
ISBN: 978-09936386-3-3 (Paperback)

www.claudettealexander.com

DEDICATION

Dedicated to my husband, Malcolm—
the wind beneath my wings.

Your love and care has propelled me to new
heights and helped me to enjoy this big,
beautiful, and wonderful world.

CONTENTS

DISCLAIMER

The author of this book do not dispense medical advice or prescribe the use of any technique as a form of treatment for physical, emotional, or medical problems without the advice of a physician, either directly or indirectly. The intent of the author is only to offer information of a general nature to help you in your quest for emotional and physical well-being. In the event you use any of the information in *A Helping Hand On Dialysis: Power Tips To Enhance The Dialysis Life* for yourself, the author nor the publisher assumes no responsibility for your actions.

"The quality of any advice anybody has to offer has to be judged against the quality of life they actually lead."

—Douglas Adams,

PREFACE

August 2003, was a turning point in my life. I began dialysis in August 2003. This resulted in a drastic change to my work, food, and lifestyle habits. My brain raced with thoughts of my mom who died from a stroke at age 48. At age 52, I wondered if it was my turn for an untimely exit. God had given me a few years more than my mom.

I reflected on the impact this would have on the lives of my two sons, one eleven and one twenty-five. My eldest son was old enough to fend for himself, but my youngest still needed his mother. I wasn't ready to die, determined to repel the Grim Reaper, should he appear. I remember tears masking my face as my outlook turned dark and gloomy, unprepared for the raging storm ahead of me.

Today, February 2015, 11 years later, I am at peace, and still hanging on. I have transitioned from fear and anxiety to calm, acceptance, and happiness. I have gained enough wisdom to share these powerful tips on enhancing the dialysis life. There have been highs, and lows, watching patients happy with their new transplanted kidney and others who leave this earth. I observed the decline in mobility when people moved from walking to cane, from cane to walker, from walker to wheelchair, and then to a motorized scooter. It was heart-wrenching.

I've seen what happens when people do not follow their healthcare professional's instructions, or cut short the duration of their dialysis regularly.

This book is intended for people on dialysis. It is mind-boggling when you are informed you need to go on dialysis to stay alive. Not all people cope in the same way to the diagnosis. Those who refused the treatment do so to their own detriment.

I hope this book will also provide comfort to the friends and family of people on dialysis, and give advice on how to support their loved ones through this medical treatment.

I hope this book will offer nuggets of information that will prove useful to anyone suffering with a chronic ailment, or to their loved ones. We all go through similar mixed emotions. Being able to manage and improve our quality of life is paramount to our happiness.

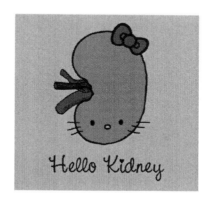

Hello Kidney

1
AN OVERVIEW

THE KIDNEYS

The kidneys are a pair of bean-shaped structures in the lower back region. Kidneys contain several functions, each one as important as the next. The main functions are:

- To filter the toxins from your blood and secrete them as urine through your bladder,
- Keep levels of electrolytes stable, such as sodium, potassium, and phosphate,

- Prevent the build-up of wastes and extra fluid in the body, and
- Make hormones that help regulate blood pressure, make red blood cells, and keep bones strong.

The average person will live a few weeks without a functioning kidney. I noticed that the people who reduce their dialysis time or skip the treatment regularly are no longer with us.

One of the major consequences of skipped treatments is difficulty breathing due to fluid build-up in the lungs. A quick test of excess fluid in the body is swelling around the ankles and wrist. Another visible sign is a dent left on the legs from wearing socks.

Dialysis or transplant might be necessary when nephrons, the filters located in your kidneys, become blocked or inflamed. As kidney function decreases, typically below 20%, doctors will advise these *renal replacement therapies* or RRTs. They are called such because the treatment works to replace the normal function of the kidneys.

There are three categories for kidney failure:

1. High blood pressure is one of the known causes of kidney failure.
2. Diabetes is another known cause.
3. Unknown.

(Note: A urine test which shows protein is an indication of a loss of kidney function. A creatinine test done through the blood, determines the percentage of function loss.)

I fall into the unknown category. Doctors cannot tell what caused my kidney failure. It could be this, or it could be that. Bottom line, they have no clue and neither do I. Long before I had high blood pressure or diabetes, I had signs of a declining kidney.

The journey of my kidney failure is detailed in my novel *Sunrise From An Icy Heart: A Memoir.*

Here is an informative video from the American National Kidney Foundation:

https://www.youtube.com/watch?v=hbwghSUW Juo

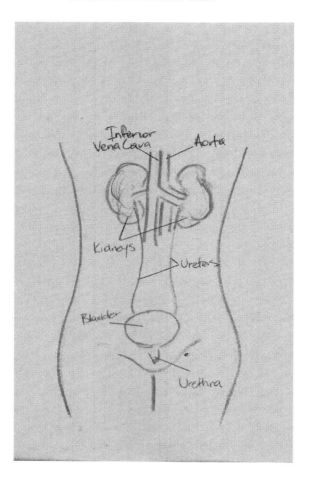

The kidneys and urinary system

KIDNEY DIALYSIS

Kidney dialysis is a life-sustaining treatment, intended to prolong life without curing or reversing the underlying kidney failure.

Kidney failure can be acute (sudden) or chronic (long-standing). Acute renal failure is a sudden loss of the kidney's ability to remove waste. It can be caused by diseases, low blood pressure because of an illness, injury, or infections. Chronic renal failure is the slow loss of kidney functions.

My loss took 21 years. (June 1982, the first sign of a problem with my kidneys to August 2003 when I went on dialysis.)

It is essential to balance your minerals while on dialysis. This is done by restricting your intake of potassium, phosphorous, and phosphate. Routine blood test determines your mineral levels. The doctor will prescribe other additional pills needed to be taken to stay in balance.

There are two types of dialysis: Peritoneal dialysis and hemodialysis.

Peritoneal dialysis

This procedure is done through the abdomen and works by gravity. A special fluid is inserted in the abdomen via a hanging tube. This fluid absorbs waste products from the blood as it passes through the peritoneum lining in the abdomen. It also removes potassium and excess fluids from the body and sends them through a tube into a bag that rest on the floor.

Peritoneal dialysis is flexible and less restrictive to location. It can be done at home or anywhere. Extreme care needs to be taken in keeping the area clean. I've done exchanges in the back seat of my car. I kept a supply of cleaning stuff in my trunk. PD users need to keep themselves in check. The dialysis fluid loses its protectiveness after four hours.

One year later, I opted to go on the *continuous cycler peritoneal dialysis, (CCPD)*. This procedure uses a machine called an 'automatic cycler' to do the exchanges every night while I slept.

One and a half years after doing peritoneal dialysis, I got an infection called peritonitis. This is an inflammation of the peritoneum, the membrane that lines part of the abdominal wall. This caused three months stay in the hospital with me fighting for survival. The Pearly Gates refused me admittance. It was not yet my time. (See Excerpt at the back of this book) After this near death scenario, I opted for hospital hemodialysis.

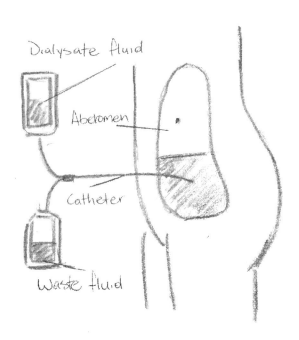

Continuous Ambulatory
Peritoneal Dialysis

Dialysate fluid

Abdomen

Catheter

Waste fluid

Hemodialysis

In this procedure, the patient is hooked up with tubes to a dialysis machine. Blood passes from the patient through a tube leading to the machine. There, the blood is cleaned and excess fluid removed. The clean blood is then returned to the patient. This is a continuous flow that lasts between three and four hours, and is done three times a week. In some cases, a session may last two hours and be done six days a week. It depends on the individual and how much kidney function is remaining.

This procedure is usually done at a dialysis center or in the hospital. Home hemodialysis has become an alternate way for patients to have the treatment without going into a centre or hospital. This is typically available after a two week training period.

In January 2015, the hospital introduced a new method of dialysis on a trial basis. The patient goes to the hospital and hemodialysis is done in the night from 8.00 P.M. The patients get a longer treatment and leaves at 6 AM. They currently operate on three shifts, 7AM, noon, and 5PM.

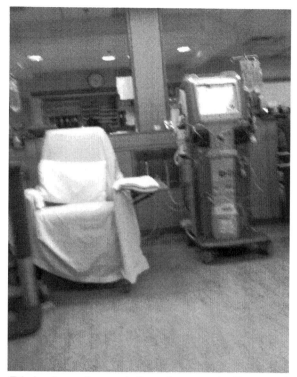

Dialysis set up at Scarborough General
Hospital, Toronto, Ontario, Canada.

I refused to try out the home hemodialysis.
One bout of peritonitis was enough to scare me
for life. I was content to show up and be
treated by the nurses. Anything could go wrong
during the treatment and I was taking no
chances. I had seen enough people pass out
during their dialysis treatment. Sometimes their
blood pressure could drop too low or problems

with the machine itself. Besides, my husband was more concerned than I, and it would not be feasible in my home. Some people do like that option. To each his own.

My kidney doctor, Dr. Ting once said, "But you did so well on the home PD before, so what's the problem?"

"That was with water Doc. This is blood."

"Well, we can change the blood to water for you."

"Ha ha. Very funny, Doc. I'll come and have my spa treatments at the hospital."

The actual process of transferring blood is not painful, but many people experience different difficulties during dialysis. Such as, cramping, low blood pressure, dizziness, and other mishaps.

Transplant

A few people bypass dialysis and head straight into transplant.

If you have someone willing to give you a kidney, and they pass the required investigative test for suitability, you may get a transplant. If not, your next choice is to wait for organ donation.

Deceased donor transplants have a long waiting list, which means you can be on the waiting list for many years before a suitable match is made for you.

A kidney transplant is not a cure, but it can improve your quality of life.

A transplanted kidney can last a few days, weeks, or years. Some people have to have several transplants in their lifetime.

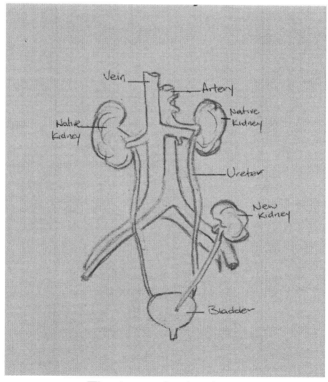

The transplant set up.

During a transplant, the old kidneys are not removed, and the new one is added in the lower abdomen.

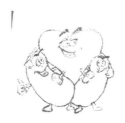

You don't understand, nor appreciate
the full functions of your kidneys
until they are no longer working.

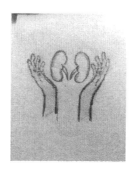

2
STARTING DIALYSIS

Before starting dialysis, there were many follow-up visits with my nephrologists (kidney doctor), followed by several blood and urine tests. Then came the day when my doctor said, "You need to go on dialysis if you want to stay alive."

I went into denial followed by a wave of emotions—fear, anxiety, anger, and many more. To get my body ready for dialysis involved a visit inside the operating room to insert tubes called catheters into my body. What the doctors did not tell me was the way I would feel after this particular operation.

I felt like my chin was clamped to my chest. A feeling that lasted a month after the get-ready-for-dialysis operation.

First, he gave me a choice—peritoneal dialysis, also known as PD or hemodialysis. He explained both dialysis procedures. At that stage the PD sounded more flexible, because I could do the procedure any place, anywhere. The hemodialysis sounded too restrictive. Who wants to go to the hospital three times a week at the same time every time? These people do not realize we have busy lives to live.

I made the decision to use the PD as my form of dialysis. There were two operations required prior to beginning my treatment. The first involved the insertion of a catheter into my abdomen, and the second, the insertion of one into my neck to begin hemodialysis temporarily while I waited for my incisions to heal. This took a month.

The procedure for inserting a hemodialysis line was not considered a drastic one, and could be carried out in the special procedure room. I was informed it was rather simple. All I needed to do was to remain still while the specialist made an incision in my neck through which to insert the tubes. I was surprised to discover he expected me to endure all this without anesthetic, nor any freezing. Heck no!

This called for some serious mouthing off to the doctor. To make matters worse he informed me he did not have all day to carry out this simple procedure.

"Simple, my ass," I responded.

I summoned all my God-given strength and lay as still as possible, long enough to get the much-needed catheter. But something had gone wrong or so I thought, because I could not remove my chin from my chest. *Relax.....this too shall pass.* It took a month for me to recover the full use of my neck. It was during those times I wondered, *is this it?* I prayed a lot and was in serious negotiations with God. Searching for any sign of death, I examined my face in the mirror, but all I saw was my blood shot eyes staring back at me.

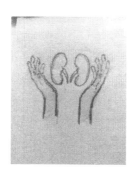

Dialysis helps to keep you alive so you can spend more time with your family and friends.

Put on your safety boots, grab a helmet and get ready as I take you on a journey with tips and strategies to enhance the dialysis life.

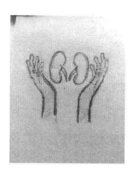

3

ON DIALYSIS

THE CLEANING SOLUTION

Two types of cleaning solution are used to clean the exit site of the catheter. One is transparent, called chlorhexidine gluconate, and the other is a brown solution, called iodine. Patients prefer the clean sight of the clear solution rather than the brown which has a messy appearance. I do not know what is in the clear solution that makes the skin around my neck itchy. After many days and weeks of scratching I realized the source came from the cleaning solution. These days I clean with the brown solution and minimize the itching.

Itching also occurs when the body has a high phosphorous level.

Tape

If you are on the peritoneal method you will use plenty of tape to hold the dressing in place.

(I'm referring to the one-inch tape). Some people are allergic to the plastic tape and have to use the paper tape. It took a lot of scratching before I figured there was a difference in the tape applied to the skin.

Many size coverings are used in the hemodialysis. Find the one that is least scratchy for you. The less scratching you do the more you can enjoy your day.

Catheters

Catheters for dialysis are in the base of my neck, near my collarbone. I had two operations to put a fistula (the joining of two veins to make a larger vein) in my left arm. They did not work. As my veins were too small. A graft (a short piece of tubing under the skin) was put into my right arm but, this did not work. Catheters in the neck are a temporary site but for me, it has become permanent.

In the beginning, I constantly explained to strangers the tubes that stuck out of my neck.

Many people are unaware about dialysis and what it entails. Sometimes, I would be in a clothing store or on the road and the site of my tubes started a discussion. I would feel embarrassed. Sometimes, I reluctantly explained my condition. I experienced different types of reactions, from alarm to sorrow for my situation. I now develop a relaxed attitude I owe no one any explanation. When strangers eye my tubes and say, "Oh my! What happened?"

"Oh! It's one of life's roadblocks," I reply with a smile.

I end the conversation right there. No further discussion needed and walk away leaving them bewildered. No need to allow them to stress me out. Life is much happier not discussing my situation. Sometimes, I use this as an opportunity to educate people, but it is not every time I am in the educating mood.

Because I am comfortable with my circumstances, I no longer go out of my way to wrap-up my neck to hide my tubes. Why should I discomfort myself so a stranger could see pleasing things? Don't look at me. Take your eyes and stare somewhere else.

I don't walk around showing. I stopped getting a headache figuring out how to hide it. I wear what I want and use scarves. If someone sees it, then so what? That is their problems not mine.

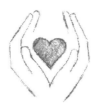

You have to find the tape or cleaning
solution that is least scratchy for you

You are the CEO of your health.
You owe it to yourself and your loved
ones to do all you can do to self-
manage your health.
Claim your power.

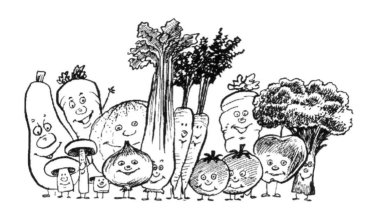

4
THE RENAL DIET

Dialysis comes with food restrictions. Since the kidneys no longer can balance minerals in the body, it has to be done manually. This is done by eating less food that has potassium, phosphorous, and phosphate and undergoing regular blood testing of these mineral levels.

The dietician connected to your program should offer a list of foods that are high, medium, and low in these minerals.

The renal diet can be dull and boring but, you do not have to let it be. Food can be fun and exciting, even when you are on a restricted diet. There are clever ways to spruce up even the blandest meal.

Things to keep in mind on the renal diet: (Talk with your nutritionist.)

1. Eat more protein. Proteins are essential for building and maintaining muscles and for the immune system to work.

2. Keep sodium low. High level of sodium can cause fluid retention.

3. Lower phosphorus intake. When the kidneys can no longer regulate the excess phosphorous in the body, you must consume less to protect your bones. Too much phosphorous in the body causes calcium to be depleted from the bones.

4. Watch potassium intake. Most of the West Indian fruits and vegetables, such as avocado, mangoes, breadfruit, soursop, tamarind, papaya, plantain, and guava are high in potassium. These foods are big struggles for me. I limit the intake and savor every morsel. High levels of potassium can affect your heart. Review your list of foods that are high, mid and low in potassium and be informed. It's okay to have one high potassium food a day. Too much of a

low potassium food can turn into a high potassium food. Watch your portion sizes.

5. Enjoy your meals. You have to be vigilant about the foods you eat when your kidneys no longer work.

6. Make your food work for you not against you. I aim for a daily mixture of seven servings of vegetables and fruits.

Patients on the peritoneal dialysis need not worry too much about potassium as some of it is lost in the drainage. They can enjoy high potassium foods. Those on the hemodialysis have to be restrictive with the intake of these minerals. Make sure you follow the dietary changes your health care team advices.

FLUIDS

Patients are weighed at every dialysis session and any increase in weight between sessions is fluid gained. Sometimes that is true and sometimes not. It means your body weight has increased.

Removal of too much fluid can cause painful cramps, and sometimes low blood pressure which could make you dizzy.

Keeping the fluid intake to a low is a big

struggle for people on dialysis. Everything has fluid—ice cream, yogurt, soups, fruits and juices. One way to reduce your water is to suck ice. A cup of ice holds less water than a cup of water.

You will feel a lot better if you try to remove two to three kilos at a time. Anything more can be stressful on the body.

SALADS

Salads are great ways to get several servings of fruits and vegetables. There are a few delicious pre-washed packaged ones at the grocery stores. The San Morino mix, baby lettuce, and spring mix are great. Check your local stores to see what selection they have. These pre-packaged ones are usually in the cooler section away from the main produce section.

I enjoy a big salad for lunch, together with a protein and a starch. Cucumbers and a fruit, such as, grapes, cherries, cranberries, and blueberries can be added to the salad for a bit of crunch. *Yummy!*

Two other pre-package vegetable salad kits which have seven super-foods I find to be nutritious are:

Sweet Kale which includes: Broccoli,

Brussels sprouts, cabbage, kale, chicory, dried cranberries, roasted pumpkin seeds, and poppy seed dressings.

Wild greens and quinoa which includes: Kale, beet greens, broccoli stalk, carrots, red cabbage, crispy quinoas, almonds, feta cheese, and avocado herb dressing.

Again, these are kept in the cooler section and not among the regular produce.

HEART HEALTHY DIET

Add Omega-3 supplements to your diet for optimal health. Kidneys and heart need all the help they can get. Omega-3 can be found in salmon, herring, krill, and flax seed. They are also found in big fat capsules. One capsule daily should help.

Here are two of my favorite homemade salads:

REGULAR SALAD FOR DINNER OR LUNCH

Ingredients:
- San Marino mix or spring mix or Baby Romaine lettuce.
- Kale, celery, grapes, blueberries, cucumber, strawberries, and tangerine.

The added fruits give the salads enough sweetness you can skip the dressing.

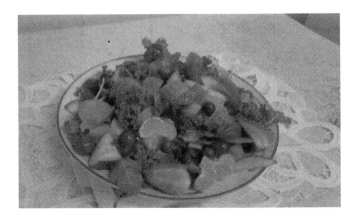

KALE SALAD FOR LUNCH
(In portable container)

Ingredients:
- Chopped kale.
- Celery, cucumber, olives, mango, strawberries, pear, and ham. (A few of each).

I do dialysis at noon so I always walk with my lunch to eat during dialysis. The kale or regular salad plus one slice bread with a protein are enough for me to eat during dialysis.

Not everybody can handle eating during

the dialysis.

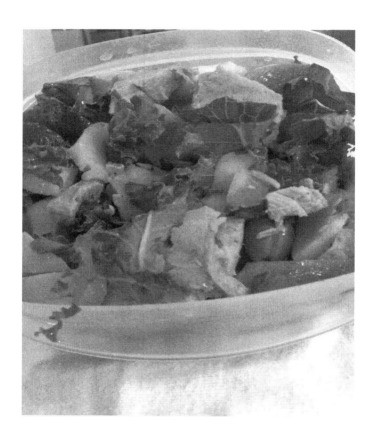

A few of the many vegetables and fruits on a renal diet.
Yummmmmmy!
(Skip the tomato)

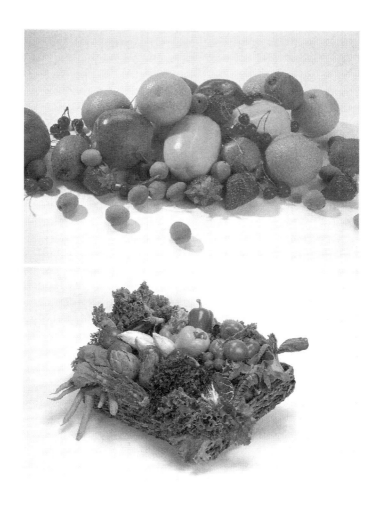

<><><>

FROM NUTRITION HANDOUTS AT THE SCARBOROUGH GENERAL HOSPITAL, CANADA

POTASSIUM FOODS

FRUITS AND VEGETABLES

 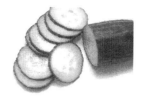

LOW POTASSIUM

JUICES: Apple juice, cranberry juice, lemon juice, lime juice, blackberry juice, and grape juice.

Nectars: apricot, guava, mango, papaya, peach, and pear.

FRUITS: Apple rings (5 dried), applesauce, blackberries, blueberries, clementine, crab-apple, cranberries, cranberry sauce, gooseberries, loganberries, mandarin, oranges (canned), pineapple, raspberries, strawberries, tangerine, watermelon, lemon, lime, and mango (1/2).

VEGETABLES: Asparagus (canned), alfalfa sprouts, bamboo shoots (canned), broccoli, cabbage, cassava, celery (raw), chayote (chocho, christophene), collards, cucumber, dandelion greens, eggplant, Belgian endive, green and yellow string beans, yellow wax beans, leeks, lettuce (all types), mushrooms (raw), onion, peppers, radish, turnip greens, water chestnuts (canned), watercress (raw),cauliflower, French green beans, eggplant, red radish, yellow squash, and Chinese broccoli.

MEDIUM POTASSIUM

JUICES: Grape juice, grapefruit juice, pineapple juice, and tangerine juice.

FRUITS: Apple, casaba melon, cherries, currant (fresh), elderberries, grapes, pear, plum, grapefruit (1/2 medium), lychees, peach, pomelo, and starfruit.

VEGETABLES: Artichoke (canned hearts), carrot, corn, kale, mushroom (canned), green peas, snow peas, spinach (raw), summer squash, zucchini, and double boiled potato (1/2 cup).

HIGH POTASSIUM

JUICES: Orange juice, passion fruit juice, prune juice, carrot juice, clamato juice, orange juice, tomato juice, vegetable juice, coconut juice/water, and V8 juice.

FRUITS: Apricots, banana, breadfruit, cantaloupe, dried fruits (all types), guava, honeydew melon, jackfruit, kiwi, mango, nectarines, orange, papaya, persimmon, pomegranate, sapodilla, soursop, coconut, dates, prunes, tamarind, and guava.

<u>VEGETABLES</u>: Artichoke (fresh), asparagus, avocado, baked beans, bamboo shoots, (fresh, boiled), dried beans/peas/lentils (examples: chick peas, lentils, split peas, kidney beans, soya beans), Brussels sprouts, bok choy, celery (boiled), Swiss chard, green banana, kohlrabi, lotus roots, mushrooms (dried/.cooked), okra, parsnips, potatoes (roasted, microwave, French fries, potato chips,), plantain, pumpkin, spinach (cooked), sweet potato, taro, tomato and tomato products, water chestnuts (fresh), winter squash (acorn, butternut, hubbard), yam, bitter melon, beet, and sweet potato.

MILK AND DAIRY PRODUCTS
LOW PHOSPHORUS

Rice Dream (Not Enriched); cream cheese.

MEDIUM PHOSPHOROUS

Custard, cream soup, ice cream, milk, pudding, sherbet, and yogurt.

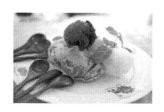

HIGH PHOSPHOROUS
Hard cheese, Evaporated milk and coffee whitener.

GRAIN PRODUCTS

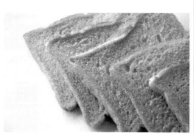
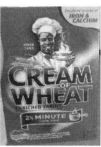

LOW POTASSIUM
BREADS: Egg bread, English muffin (plain), Italian bread, light rye, reduced calorie oat bran, reduced calorie oatmeal, reduced calorie rye, reduced calorie wheat, reduced calorie white, roll- 60% whole wheat, white bread, white pita, sourdough bread, breadstick, cracked wheat, hamburger bun, hot dog bun, Kaiser bun, plain white bagel, and white roti.

CERERALS (COLD): Cheerios, corn bran, cornflakes, crispix, crispy rice, Kashi puffed, puffed rice, puffed wheat, rice krispies, and special k.

CEREALS (HOT): Cornmeal porridge, cream of rice, cream of wheat, farina, and wheatlets.

RICE/PASTA/GRAINS: White rice, white pasta, egg noodles, rice noodles, and soba noodles.

CRACKERS Cream crackers, graham crackers, Melba toast, rice cakes, soda crackers, taco/tortilla shell, and water crackers.

BAKED GOODS: Arrowroot cookies, Angel food cake, homemade muffins, oatmeal cookies, pound cake, short bread cookies, and social tea biscuits.

HIGH POTASSIUM

BREADS: Cornbread, cracked wheat, English muffin, multigrain, pumpernickel, raisin bread, rice bran bread, whole wheat bread, whole wheat pita, wheat bran, wheat germ, and oatmeal bread.

CEREALS (COLD): All bran, all bran buds, 100% bran, bran flakes, cheerios (multigrain), fibre 1, fruit & fibre (all varieties), just right, oat bran, oat squares, raisin bran, shreddies, wheatbix, granola, grape nuts, honey nut cheerios, life cereal, and puffed wheat.

CEREALS: Bulgur, Maltex, and oatmeal

RICE/PASTA/GRAINS: Whole grain pasta, whole grain rice, wild rice, oat cakes, bran muffin, pancake, waffle, and whole grain roll.

BAKED GOODS: Chocolate coated cookies, peanut butter sandwich cookies,

cookies with lots of nuts,and muffins,

CRACKERS: Cheddar cheese-flavored crackers, crackers with peanut butter or cheese filling, milk crackers, rye and whole grain crackers, triscuits, and crackers with seeds.

OTHER ITEMS
LOW POTASSIUM

Mayonnaise, sugar, jelly, jams, margarine, butter, coffee, tea, lemonade, and fruit punch.

HIGH POTASSIUM

Nuts and seeds, coconut in any form, chocolate, potato chips, brown sugar, molasses, maple sugar or maple syrup, specialty coffee (example cappuccino, espresso, Turkish coffee) cocoa, and Ovaltine.

PHOSPHOROUS
CHOOSE:

Plain bagels, cracked wheat bread, croissant, crumpets, English muffin, French, Italian, Kaiser roll, raisin bread, taco shell, white bread, and white pita.

Corn bran, corn chex, corn flakes, cornmeal, cream of rice, cream of wheat, grits, puffed rice, rice krispies, rice flakes, Applejacks, captain crunch, crispix, Froot loops, and honeycomb.

Melba toast, unsalted soda crackers, Angel food cake, arrowroot, fruit pies, pound cake, puff pastry, shortbread, social tea, sponge cake, white pasta, white rice, yeast donuts, Cake, muffins, pancakes and waffles made with baking powder.

Meat/fish/poultry, low sodium cold cuts, shrimp, lobster, crabs, tofu, natural hard cheese, egg, and peanut butter.

All fruits and vegetables.

All soft drinks.

Cream, custard, ice cream, milk and anything made with milk such as pudding and cream soup, sherbet, and yogurt.

AVOID:

Whole grain breads—bran, cornbread, dark rye, multigrain, scone, tortilla, and whole wheat.

Wholegrain cereals—Alphabits, bran, buckwheat, bulger, cheerios, granola, grape nuts, life, muesli, oatmeal, puffed wheat, raisin bran, shredded wheat, special k, and weetabix.

Rye and whole grain crackers, brown rice, barley, buckwheat, bulger, cake, donuts, wild rice, pies or pastries made with nuts, chocolate, cream or custard. Most commercial cookies.

Caviar, fish roe oyster, Clams, mussels, scallops, bones (canned sardines/salmon), liver, brain, kidney, all dried beans, peas & lentils, and process cheese.

Ovaltine, malted milk, Mylo, Horlicks, chocolate, cola products, beer, nuts & seeds.

Chocolate milk, ice cream with chocolate or nuts.

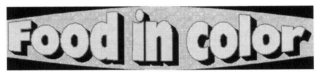

Think about food in colors. Add a variety of color when you eat your vegetables and fruits. Here are examples for eating in colors:

- ████—to improve heart and blood health.
  Red leaf lettuce, radishes, red peppers, red cherries, red apples, and pink grapefruits, strawberries, watermelon, raspberries, and cranberries.
- Orange—to prevent inflammation.
  Carrots, pumpkin, sweet potatoes, butternut squash, tangerines, and peaches.
- Purple—to protect the nervous system.
  Eggplant, red cabbage, grapes, and blueberries.

- **Yellow**—to fortify skin elasticity. Corn, summer squash, lemon, pineapple, and golden apples.
- White—to strengthen the immune system. Cauliflower, garlic, mushroom, pear, and white grapefruit.
- ▮▮▮▮▮—to detoxify. Lettuce and leafy greens (collards, kale, arugula, dandelions, watercress, spinach), broccoli, cucumbers, snow peas, green beans, okra, green grapes, limes, green apples, and green plums.

Those patients with the combos (kidney failure and diabetes) need not only have to be aware of the renal diet, but also be conscious of the glucose content of foods. Most people know what they should be eating. Most often the problem is not what they are eating, but how much of it. Portion control is something many people have to consider when planning their meals. Many are more comfortable with visuals. Another alternative to measuring is to use your hands to estimate your portion size. A method I find to be very useful.

Handy portion guide

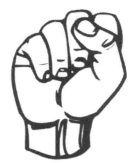

FRUITS/GRAINS & STARCHES

Choose an amount the size of your fist for each of grains and starches, and fruit.

VEGETABLES

Choose as much as you can hold in both hands.

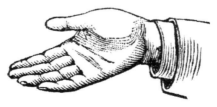

MEAT AND ALTERNATIVES

Choose an amount up to the size of the palm of your hand and the thickness of your little finger.

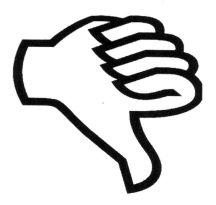

FATS
Limit fat to an amount the size of the tip of your thumb.

MILK AND ALTERNATIVES
Drink up to 250 ml (8 oz) of low-fat milk or alternatives with a meal.

From Meal Planning for Healthy Eating Diabetes Prevention and Management, Canadian Diabetes Association. http://www.diabetes.ca/diabetes-and-you/healthy-living-resources/diet-nutrition/portion-guide

CLAUDETTE ALEXANDER

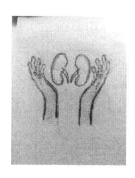

Make your food work for you, not against you.

If you are on an airplane and it's going down you are advised to put the oxygen mask on yourself first before you can help anybody else.
In other words take care of yourself first, then you will be able to help other people.

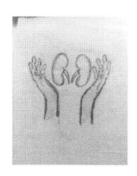

5
SUPPORT SYSTEM

It can be emotionally and physically challenging when you are diagnosed with a chronic illness. It helps to have a support system in place. A support system can be a spouse, children, family and friends, or even support groups.

Feeling supported is essential to human life. Nourishment comes not only from food and water, but also from connecting to others. I am full of gratitude for Magic Jack, A **device that plugs into a computer and allows the user to make free long distance calls,** and the Internet.

They allow me to talk with long distance family and friends.

Support systems are special gifts to be cherished and enjoyed. They offer the following;

- A listening ear.
- A feeling you are cared and supported.
- Help through bumps on the road.
- Comfort when needed.

My support system comprises of my husband, children, grandchildren, siblings, and a few friends. They keep me laughing and enjoying life.

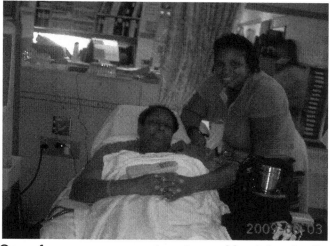

One of my many support systems: My sister, Lydia, who always has my back. At Scarborough General Hospital, Scarborough, Ontario, Canada

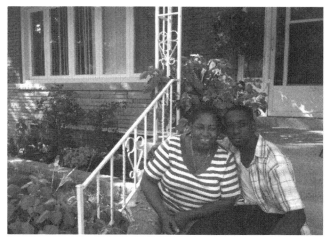

One of my support systems: My son, Kriston, who ensures the exterior of my home stays beautiful.

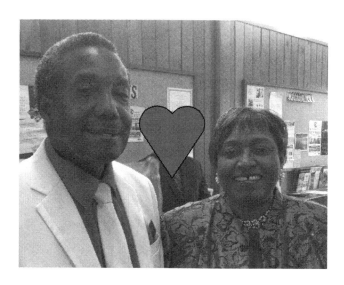

One of my support systems: My husband, Malcolm, who keeps me smiling.

Facebook has many support groups. A few I belong to include:

- Living With Kidney Failure – End Stage Renal Disease (ESRD) Support Group
- Kidney Disease, Dialysis, and transplant.
- I Hate Dialysis. (Don't let the name fool you. They are not negative, but rather supportive.)

Don't go it alone. Build your support system. It will make the journey more bearable, help with living happy with chronic conditions and it may extend your life.

For residents of Canada:

The Kidney Foundation of Canada has a Peer Support Program which allows you to speak to someone. Their brochure can be downloaded:

The Kidney Connect Peer
Support Program'
http://www.kidney.ca/document.doc?id=4394

or they can be reached by phone at
1-866-390-7337.

For residents of the United States:

https://www.kidney.org/patients/peer
855-NKF-PEER (855-653-7337) or

EMAIL: NKFPEERS@KIDNEY.ORG

For all other worldwide residents:
Check the Kidney Foundation of your local state for a Peer Support Program.

"Whether or not you have a supportive community of friends and family, one thing you do have on your side is life. Part of reconnecting is knowing that life loves you. Life has your back. When you trust life to support you, you are never alone. Life will always support you as you take the power of your health and happiness back into your own hands."

Loving Yourself To Great Health
By
Louise Hay,
Ahlea Khadro,
and Heather Dane

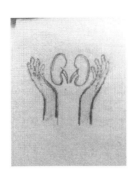

Support systems are special gifts to
be cherished and enjoyed.

"I observe with joy as life abundantly supports and cares for me."

------Loving Yourself To Great Health

by
Louise Hay, Ahlea Khadro, and Heather Dane

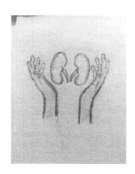

6
DIALYSIS AND SEX

Dialysis does not lower your libido. Maybe, at first, but as long as blood runs through your veins, you got to have it when you want it. For those with a catheter in their abdomen for the PD dialysis then roast chicken style (missionary position) is just out of the question. You certainly do not want anyone pressing on your vital catheter. Besides, the fullness of your stomach from all that dialysis fluid stored in there renders that action not very pleasurable.

Get creative folks. I am not suggesting that you become an acrobat or you get into 101 ways to please your lover. If you are young, go for it, but if you are like me, hitting the sixties, I need to lie down. Can't stand up and touch my toes. I would surely fall over and damage my catheter. If you have ever had a colonoscopy, you will get the drift. For those who haven't and are still waiting for the big bang just lie on your side in the fetal position and get your action.

People who are on hemodialysis, need not worry about catheter in their stomach, but rather the one in the neck. You can enjoy your roast chicken style, but you still need to worry that in the heat of the action, your neck catheter does not get ripped off. Go for the colonoscopy style.

Those who do dialysis through the arm, then by all means go for your avalanche of throbbing pleasure any way you want. But wait, you have to worry about putting too much weight on your arm, hence you do the balancing act.

Now, let us not forget that love making is not only penetration. Intimacy, giving each other a little massage to soothe the aching body, holding hands, taking small or long walks, dancing, laughing together, talking to each other or doing the dishes. Other loving gestures include accompanying your partner to dialysis sessions occasionally, making or buying a meal and having it waiting after dialysis. Whatever works with your budget and time.

Some people may have a reduced libido, but I think it has more to do with the aging process as opposed to the dialysis.

In any case, if you cannot get your freak on, you should consult your doctor.

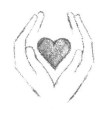

Love making is not only penetration.

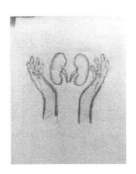

7
CRAMPING

One of the many functions of the kidneys is to remove excess fluid from the body. When that function is gone, you may experience weight gain from excess fluid between dialysis treatments. This excess is removed during dialysis. Cramping occurs when too much fluid is removed. Too much fluid in the body causes difficulty in breathing because the excess fluid goes to the lungs.

The way to avoid cramping is to not remove too much fluid or not to drink too much. When one has gained weight instead of just extra fluid, and too much fluid is removed during the dialysis, then this can cause cramping. Some patients make the mistake of wanting more fluid removed, refusing to accept the fact that they have gained weight. (Keep in mind this is not a diet and removing more fluid than necessary is not the way to lose weight).

Doctors advised their dialysis patients to remove less than 2 kg of fluid during the week and less than 3 kg on weekends. This is difficult as foods that melt (such as ice cream, frozen treats, juices, ice) and foods that contain liquids (such as soup) are all classed as liquids. This means, one has to be vigilant with fluid intake. I find that when I stay within those margins of fluid removal my body recovers much better after dialysis and I don't get that *run-down* feeling. When I remove over 3 kg, then I get wasted for the rest of the day. When I get home, I lie on the couch and sleep while watching television.

Many years ago, I attended a Kidney Symposium put on by The Kidney Foundation of Ontario. We had fun workshops and learned a great deal of useful information on the kidneys and other resources available to patients. We sang a cramping song, and it has remained with me.

This song is sang to the tune of "Are you Lonesome tonight" By Elvis Presley

<u>ARE YOU CRAMPING TONIGHT</u>

Are you cramping tonight?
Are your muscles uptight?
Are you sad that your kidneys have failed?
Does your memory stray to those more healthy days when you could drink as much as you pleased?
Do you sit by your loved ones who helplessly care?
Do you try not to bug them when they see you there?
Is your life different now?
Have you less fun somehow?
Tell me dear, are you cramping tonight?

—(Unknown)

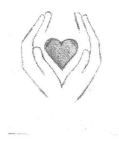

Be vigilant with your fluid intake.

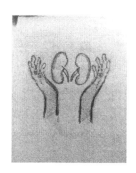

8
MUSIC THERAPY

A few years ago, I used to go to a music therapy session with a group of dialysis patients at a place called Carefirst. It was a fun activity, and we created a few songs of our own. Our instructor used a guitar, and we composed the songs. Sometimes, we just sang a variety of songs. Music therapy is another way to take your mind off the pain and problems.

The company no longer has that program, but the songs still lingers. Sadly, a few in the group who composed this song have passed. Try to find a music therapy group in your area. It can be lots of fun.

Here is one of the songs we composed:

FAITH (The Dialysis Dream Song)

If I can see, if I can feel, If I can walk.
If I can hear, if I can pray, if I can talk.
I can be grateful.
I am brand new today, yesterday can slip away.
And tomorrow will be another day.

First I felt alone and rejected.
Hopeless and abandoned and without any hope.
Now I'm renewed with love and understanding.
Today I can see, I had to reach out.
Open up my hand.
I had the faith, and I believed.
Now I can love myself as I love others.
And receive their love and care.

If I can see, if I can feel, if I can walk.
If I can hear, if I can pray, if I can talk.
I can be grateful.
I am brand new today, yesterday can slip

away.
And tomorrow will be another day.

Thank God for everything, just the way it is.
I can count my blessings, I have more than
so many.
Life has been tough, but struggle made me
strong.
Good things like family, good things like
friends.
I see the beauty in all creation.
Today I can smile.

If I can see, If I can feel, if I can walk.
If I can hear, if I can pray, if I can talk.
I can be grateful.
I am brand new today, yesterday can slip
away.
And tomorrow will be another day.

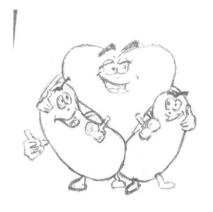

Music therapy is another way to take
your mind off the pain and difficulties
that you go through.

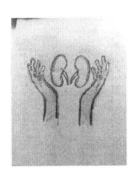

9
TRAVEL

Last minute packages which offer deep discounts on vacation travels are not for dialysis patients so there is no need to feel left out. You deal with what you have. First, you are required to be in a stable condition because no dialysis center wants to care for you with other medical complications. You need to be free of HIV, hepatitis, heart problems, and other serious medical ailments. They prefer to attend to dialysis patients who do not have many issues. Your local unit will take you with additional health issues, but the transient locations won't.

The transient center will require your dialysis centre to fax them up to date information about your current state of health. This means you need to be tested a month or two in advance of your trip. You are well aware how slow the process of getting and transmitting information from the hospital.

A standard request from a dialysis unit will ask for your current medical history, physical report, and blood work comprising of:

- Renal profile (Test about kidney function. Checks for levels of creatinine, calcium, sodium, chloride, carbon dioxide, albumin, blood urea nitrogen, protein, phosphorous, glucose, and potassium in the blood.)
- CBC (Complete blood count.)
- INR (International normalized ratio— blood clot information)
- hepatitis
- MRSA (bacteria testing of nose, exit sites, and anus.)
- Dialysis prescription
- Most recent EKG (Electrocardiogram— heart testing)
- Last three dialysis treatment sheets
- List of all current medications

Make sure you know the name of the nurse in charge and her phone and fax number. You will provide all this information to your unit and do a follow-up to see if the hospital has forwarded all your information. Confirm the receiver has all they required. Use email for out of country or city trips.

Keep on top of things and find out if your unit forwarded all the requested information. In most cases, nephrologists at the other end will review the information received and give the go ahead for you to come in.

Now your bags are packed, and you are ready to leave on your long awaited vacation. Double and triple check you have all your required medications. Ensure there are sufficient amounts to last the duration of your trip. Hemodialysis patients carry a cooler with their Erythropoietin (Epo) in it. This is an expensive medication given free of charge in Canada for patients who need it. Those with a catheter in their neck should ensure to bring extra dressing in case there is a mishap between treatments.

If you are on peritoneal dialysis (PD), you are well-aware advance arrangements need to be made with your dialysis supplier to either provide you with all the necessary fluids and supplies or have it waiting for you at your destination.

Take no chances with your medications if traveling by air. Put your medications and Epo in your carry-on bag. You don't want to reach your destination and find your luggage has gone astray for a day or two, or even longer.

If you live in Canada, you are one of the fortunate ones. Dialysis is expensive. It is a free treatment in Canada, if you have a valid Ontario Hospital Insurance Plan (OHIP).If you are vacationing within Canada, your OHIP card will be sufficient to get treatment free of charge. If you are vacationing in the United States, you would need to call the center to find out the prices. In the West Indian Islands, like St. Lucia, Barbados, Jamaica, Trinidad, etc. one treatment can cost up to US$320.00. A two week vacation with three treatments a week can run you US$1,920.00.

Your dialysis center should have a list of dialysis centers all over the world. You can also go on the website: http://globaldialysis.com/ for a wealth of information including address and phone numbers of over 161 worldwide dialysis centers. In Canada, OHIP will reimburse you CA$210.00 per dialysis treatment when you get back. It is imperative that you get a detailed statement if you want to get your refund from the OHIP office. For example, you cannot submit a bill for $2,000.00 for dialysis treatment. Your bill should include the individual dates on which you received treatment. Otherwise, if you send one bill with one amount, you are just going to get reimbursed for CA$210.00, the maximum payable by OHIP.

On one of my vacations, I traveled to Trinidad and St. Lucia and to avoid any confusion with my payment, I purchased five international money orders and paid by credit card for the sixth treatment, collecting a single bill for each treatment. In the Caribbean Islands, you pay before treatments, so make sure your credit cards are problem free if you plan on paying by credit. Money first, then dialyze.

In Canada, if you need assistance with dialysis payments, arrangements can be made well in advance for a medical loan from the Kidney Foundation of Canada. Loans of up to six treatments can be obtained equivalent to the amount OHIP will reimburse you. For example: In the Islands, each dialysis treatment is US$320.00. If you receive dialysis treatment three times a week for two weeks, you would need to pay US$1,920.00 for the six treatments (2011 prices).

OHIP will reimburse you CA$210.00 x 6 which is equal to $1,260.00.You can get a loan from the Kidney Foundation for CA$1,260.00 payable in four to five months. You should have received your payment from OHIP or assigned the refund directly to the Kidney Foundation.

Speak with your social worker at your center to see what kind of assistance is offered to dialysis patients from the Kidney Foundation in your area.

You will need to factor in transportation cost to and from dialysis when figuring out your vacation budget. In Ontario, dialysis patients have access to Wheel-Trans, which is a special transportation for people with disabilities. If you do not use a wheelchair or a motorized scooter, then regular taxis are sent to pick and drop you off when the need arises. You pay the same fare as going on the bus or train. You can arrange to be on a fixed prearranged booking, or you can call the day before to book for the next day.

I traveled to Halifax and had difficulty arranging transportation pick up and drop off. The Wheel-Trans service requires an advance booking of one week. There's no guarantee you will get a ride. It is difficult to book one week in advance if you are on vacation because the dialysis center schedules your time slot at all times of the day. They may schedule you during the morning, afternoon, or evening shift. Sometimes, you wait until the last session to find out what your time is for the next session. When you do not have a ride, then you have to either take a taxi or get someone to drop you off and pick you up.

Once you get over all your hurdles, you arrange your sightseeing around your appointments, enjoy the local cuisine and have a fantabulous time.

If you don't want to fly and would rather sail the big ocean, there are dialysis cruises which you can take that cater to dialysis patients. Dialysis is done on the ship with physicians and nurses to look after your needs. These are pricey, but if you can afford it, then by all means, set sail.

If you would rather have a camping trip, that can also be arranged. Each hospital in my area is allowed one week at a camp called Lions Camp Dorset, in Dorset, Ontario. The cottages are reasonable. I spent one week with my family at Lions Camp Dorset. We had lots of fun as I could play tennis, board games, and even sit in the kayak while my brother or son paddled. It was refreshing to be in touch with nature, take leisure walks, and just be away from the city with its hustle and bustle.

Don't deprive yourself because you are on dialysis. Get out there and enjoy yourself by land, sea, or air. Whatever your budget allows.

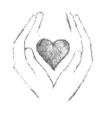

Forget about last minute vacation packages and there is no need to feel left out.

AT TAPION HOSPITAL
CASTRIES, ST. LUCIA

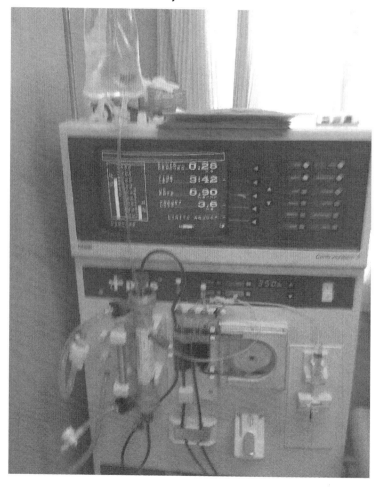

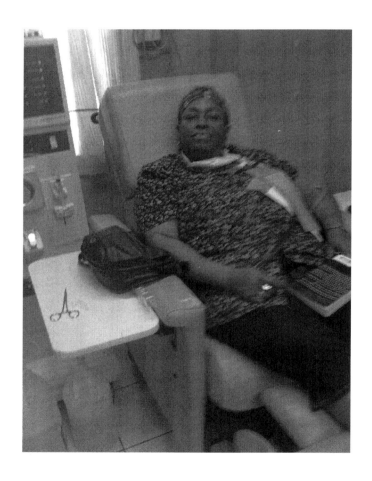

AT DARTMOUTH HOSPITAL
NOVA SCOTIA, CANADA

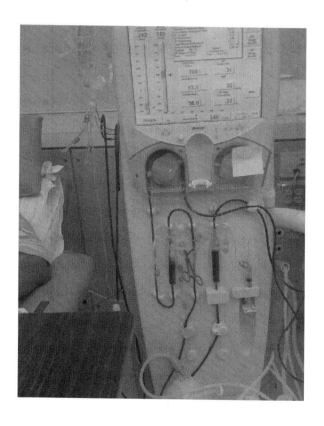

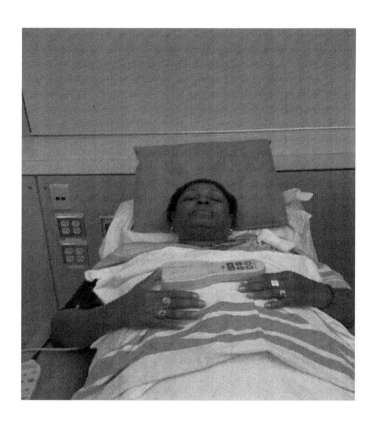

"Life can be wildly tragic at times, and I've had my share. But whatever happens to you, you have to keep a slightly comic attitude. In the final analysis, you have got to not forget to laugh."

—Katharine Hepburn

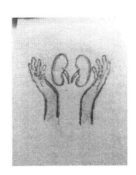

10
LAUGH FOR GOOD HEALTH

I'm sure you've heard the saying many times that laughter is the best medicine. Whatever illness you are going through, why not try a little laughter for a change? It will make you feel a whole lot better. Five compelling reasons:

1. It's free. Yes, it cost zero dollars.

2. It's healthy, you don't need any pills.

3. It feels good, and makes you forget about whatever pain you're going through.

4. Everybody speaks the language of laughter, so there's, no need to translate and.

5. You get facial exercises. So get ready and pucker up your face for a good laugh.

All together: Screw the corners of your mouth up towards your eyes and hold that pose for 30 seconds. Feel foolish? Good. Keep smiling. Permit yourself a tiny chuckle. Crack right up and let it out. Laugh until your belly bursts. Laugh till tears run from your eyes. Laugh till you can laugh no more.

Alright! Alright! Alright! If you don't want to laugh, then smile. Maybe you don't want to show your crooked teeth. Whatever?

I am always smiling or laughing. It is unusual for anybody to see me with a sad face. I recognize the comedy in everything. I love comedy, and watch them at concerts and TV.

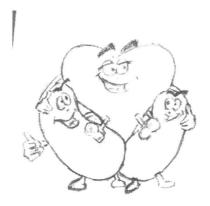

Laughter will help you feel a whole lot better

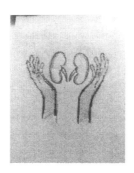

11
MEMORY BANK

Now that I am into my sixties, my body is going downhill. I do not understand whoever said we age gracefully. There's nothing graceful about using a cane to balance your aching body.

I decided from now on to take a different approach.

Since being on dialysis, I valued each day I was granted another day to enjoy this beautiful world. Instead of mourning for the parts of my body that no longer work as well, I now accept my gift of another brand new day and rejoice at the parts that are still working.

Like I enjoy my beautiful heart which still

pumps blood through my veins. Gorgeous eyes used to feast on nature and its surrounding beauty. A mind still intact. Pearly whites to chew food to nourish my body, instead of being fed through a tube, and the ability to still do number two without help or attachments to my body.

I reminisce about the happy memories the non-working parts have given me and I deposit additional happy memories into the memory banks of my mind so I can make withdrawals when I need them.

I use these five simple rules to be happy (Author unknown)

1. Free your heart from hatred.
2. Free your mind from worries.
3. Live simply.
4. Give more.
5. Expect less.

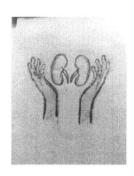

I value each and every day I have been
granted another day to enjoy this
beautiful world.

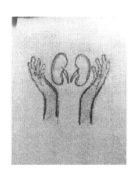

12
EXERCISE

Exercise is good for you, but when you are ill or in pain, the last thing you want to do is to move around.

Many years ago, I used to exercise and be physically active. Since I have been on dialysis, my exercise level has dropped significantly. Dialysis tires me out. On dialysis days, exercise is out of the question. I only have the energy to head to the couch and sleep. Also, my knees hurt to the point I need a cane to walk.

The day I found myself using the cane

inside my home and dragging my feet to move from one couch to the other, I knew the time had come to take this thing called exercise more seriously.

I joined a gym. This time, I made use of it, unlike earlier times when I joined and went once every three months. I got on the stationary bike and did fifteen minutes of bicycling, plus one minute on the elliptical machine, three times a week.

I gradually increased my time on the machines. Now, one year later, I am up to 35 minutes on the bike and 10 to 15 minutes on the elliptical. I have also added a weekly one hour session of chair yoga on Tuesdays, and one hour osteo fitness on Thursdays to my routine. Sometimes, I try some arm and leg machines in the gym using the lowest weight level.

There has been a vast improvement in my mobility. I walk freely in my home and outside, if I'm going short distances. I use the cane if the walk is a bit far.

You do not need to run a marathon to exercise. There are three kinds of exercise useful to the body. Twenty to thirty minutes a session, three times a week is enough to get the heart pumping, and the muscles toned.

Flexibility exercises

Long stretches loosen the muscles and joints. They help with balance and coordination. I do these while watching TV or first thing in the morning when I get out of bed.

Strength exercises

These are to strengthen my muscles. I use elastic bands and small weights. In the gym, I use arm and leg machines. Nothing strenuous. Just the first level on the weights.

Endurance or aerobic exercises

Endurance, or aerobic, activities are a little tougher than the others. Improved endurance makes it easier to carry out many everyday activities, but, you should tailor your exercise choices to your abilities.

I'm slower than I used to be and have a catheter in my neck that must stay dry, so I chose an elliptical machine over swimming and a stationary bike over walking. I can still handle some moves on the dance floor with lots of rest between these moves.

Keep in mind that swimming is a low-impact exercise that's gentle on the joints.

Other wonderful exercises

Chair yoga: One hour of arm and leg

stretches sitting on a chair. Plus neck ones.

Osteo Fitness: A half hour of marching, leg raises, kicking, and arm movements. The second half of the hour can be spent sitting on a chair doing arm and leg movements using weights, elastic bands, sticks and tennis balls.

These two exercises are so good for the arms and legs.

Michelle Obama came out with a simple and effective exercise program with her 2015 'Let's Move' campaign. Take a look at her video here:

https://youtu.be/MkHNK406BrM

I reached the stage when I could no longer stretch to my back to button my bra. I solved that problem by tacking my bra at the front and swinging it to the back. Another reason you need to work on your backstretch is because you do not want to be in the uncomfortable position of not being able to wipe after you doo-doo. Calling someone to finish the wiping job for you is certainly not sexy.

Exercise releases endorphins, and now that it is a regular part of my living, it adds to my happiness consumption: 120 plus minutes a week and I feel fantastic.

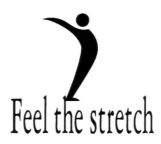

Feel the stretch

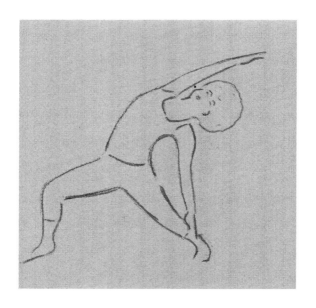

You do not need to run a marathon to exercise.

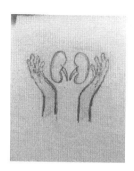

13
CHANGES

November is the final month of autumn and as the cool air begins to change and get colder, we anticipate the winter breeze. In winter, we look forward to spring and relief from the snow. In spring, we long for more comfort and cannot wait for the hot air of summer.

As nature changes with the seasons so do our lives. Each season brings its own treasures.

- Spring heralds newness—new flowers, new buds on fruit trees, and plants.
- Summer gives us time to rest, relax,

and enjoy our gardens.

- Nature puts on a show in autumn as we feast our eyes on a rainbow of colors.
- Winter brings the holidays, a time for celebration and family gatherings.

In the same way our bodies change as we get older, it is necessary to take heed of the subtle warning signs our body sends out and embrace the changes. For example, if you constantly have a headache, it is your body telling you that something is wrong. You need to check it out. Ignoring the warning signs only leads to complications down the road.

Dialysis brings changes to your lifestyle. Accept the changes, manage them, and get ready for another brand new day. Stop being in denial. Try to learn and heed the changes. No need to be slipping into a depression. Get professional help if you must. Life is too beautiful to wallow into self-pity.

"Change is the natural law of my life.
I welcome change
I am willing to change.
I choose to change my thinking.
I move from the old to the new with
ease and with joy.
I am learning to choose to make today
a pleasure to experience.
All is well in my world."

You Can Heal Your Life
By Louise L Hay

*As nature changes with the seasons so
do our lives
Embrace the changes.*

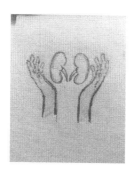

14
WORLD KIDNEY DAY

World Kidney Day is celebrated the second Thursday in March.

Celebrate the good years your kidneys gave you. Read, educate, and learn about the kidneys. You will miss them when they are gone. Mine gave me 52 good years before they said, "Adios."I surely miss their functions, but a dialysis machine helps me out now. Hugs, hugs, hugs to my machine.

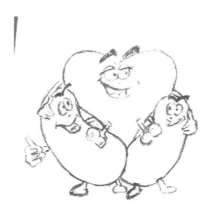

Celebrate the good years your
kidneys gave you

"Rise above the storm and you will find the sunset."

—Mario Fernandez

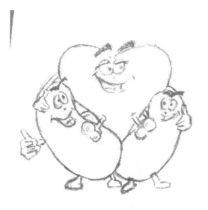

15

Inspirational Stories

When you are a dialysis patient, you can go through a wide range of emotions in a single day. Sometimes, you're up. Sometimes, you're down. Other times, you are extremely tired, and the only thing left to do is sleep.

I have had many of those days, but every so often, I read a story of someone who is in

119

worse shape than I am, yet they lead a full life. Their stories give me hope and inspiration. I hope their stories will do the same for you. Here are a few of my inspirational heroes.

Nick Vujicic

Born Nicholas James Vujicic on December 4, 1982 in Australia. No arms, no feet and yet he can do many things that the ordinary man cannot do and more. He swims, golfs, types, sky dives, cooks, and faces life with confidence.

There are many YouTube videos about him. I like this one about when he found true love:

https://www.youtube.com/watch?v=s3QezBvN1BE

Here's another video that gives an insight to his beginnings. It is one to make you forget about any problems you are going through:

The Man Who Leads With No Limbs
https://www.youtube.com/watch?v=meT-XgQix6w

His website:
http://www.lifewithoutlimbs.org/

Richie Parker

Born May 1983 in South Carolina, U.S.A. with no arms. Richie drives his big Impala and works as an engineer at NASCAR Racing Team. He use his feet to do all that his hands cannot do. He rides a bike, cooks, uses a computer, and drives a car with his feet. Richie Parker's story gives me strength.

https://www.youtube.com/watch?v=UCtIX-WWUrY

http://www.autoblog.com/2013/08/22/richie-parker-nascar-no-arms-video/

Ben Underwood

Born January 1992 in California, USA. Although Ben was born with sight, he lost it to cancer at age two. He did not let his blindness prevent him from doing anything nor did it prevent him from getting around.

The Boy Who Sees Without Eyes makes for super interesting viewing.

https://www.youtube.com/watch?v=AiBeLoB6CKE

In January 2009, the cancer took Ben's life at age 16, but his short life is still an inspiration to many.

Chris Farmer

A farmer at Apricot Lane Farms in Moorpark, California, with no arms and no legs, but he still gets the job done on the farm. Chris operates a tractor, rides a skateboard, writes, and much more. Another true inspiration:

https://www.youtube.com/watch?v=H9S3n_tILKo#t=124

Joanne O. Riorden

Born in Ireland in 1996 with a rare condition known as Total Amelia which means she has no limbs. That has not stopped Joanne from using technology to help her navigate the world around her. Truly uplifting.

https://www.youtube.com/watch?v=FQPR0pfCMx4
http://www.thejournal.ie/no-limbs-no-limits/news/

Miriam Njeru

A Kenyan mother with no arms, yet she takes care of her baby effortlessly. She cooks, washes, nurses her baby and does everything with her feet. When you see a person like

Miriam Njeru, you just have to shut your mouth and deal with your problems.

https://youtu.be/Me7x0xaGmrl

Bill Peckham

I came across Bill Peckham, who has dialyzed in 22 countries and five continents. He enjoys his vacations. One of his trips was to the Grand Canyon where he used a generator to power his dialysis. He is an inspiration to all dialysis travelers.

Check his blog: **Dialysis from the sharp end of the needle**

http://www.billpeckham.com/from_the_sharp_end_of_the/

"Life is ten percent what happens to you and 90 percent how you respond to it."

—Lou Holtz

RESOURCES

Dialysis Patient Citizens
   http://dialysispatients.org/advocacy/key-issues

Transplant Living
   http://www.transplantliving.org/

The Kidney Foundation of Canada
   http://kidney.ca/

Global Dialysis
   http://www.globaldialysis.com/

Dialysis at Sea
   http://www.dialysisatsea.com/

St. Lucia Vacation Dialysis
   http://www.stlucia-dialysis.com/

Lions Camp Dorset
   http://www.lionscampdorset.on.ca/

Dialysis Centers
   http://www.dialysiscenters.org/ (Search by
Zip Code, State or name)

The National Kidney Foundation (USA)
   https://www.kidney.org/

American Kidney Fund
   http://www.kidneyfund.org/

The American Kidney Fund has several
assistance programs to help dialysis patients.
Help can include payment of health insurance
premiums, and other treatment-related
expenses. If you are a patient who is in need of
treatment-related financial assistance, speak
with your dialysis center social worker about
submitting an application to AKF.

EXCERPT FROM:

SUNRISE FROM AN ICY HEART: A MEMOIR

BY
CLAUDETTE ALEXANDER

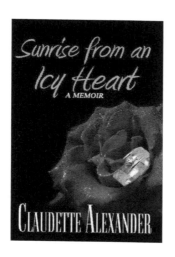

Sunrise from An Icy Heart has a grand

romance, passion and understanding that took 43 years to develop. Includes a single mother's struggles to raise sons with strong loving hearts and her battle with chronic kidney failure. In addition, it envelopes all that is special about St. Lucia, its people, and culture.

Available at retailers and online stores in paperback, Kindle and e-pub versions.

CHAPTER 51
BATTLING KIDNEY FAILURE

2003

On August 14, 2003, Canada and the United States experienced a massive blackout. Two days later the lights came back on, and then I experienced my own personal blackout. After several years of having tests done to check my creatinine levels, potassium, and protein, Dr. Ting advised me to cut down on protein, eat one chicken leg not two, increase potassium levels, and eat bananas, etc. I arrived for my usual two months' test, sat down, and waited for the results of the last test.

"Your creatinine is too high; you need to go

on dialysis to stay alive," said Dr. Ting. Your kidneys are operating at below 20 per cent, and you can no longer depend on your kidneys for survival. You need a kidney transplant."

I gripped the arm rest tightly. My mind raced. *Am not ready to die, Lord Jesus, help me.*

"Doctor, get me on the transplant list now so I can get a kidney next week."

"It does not work like that. You would have to be on the kidney transplant waiting list for five to 10 years before you can get one."

He scribbled some notes in my file.

"Why do I have to wait that long, Dr. Ting? You know I need it now. Can you tell the transplant people that I cannot wait that long? Anyway, Dr. Ting what caused my kidneys to get to below 20 per cent?"

I shifted restlessly in my chair. Over the years doctors had told me they could not pinpoint the exact cause of my kidney failure, but this time I still hoped to get a different answer.

"You have a condition called FSGS, focal segmental glomerulsclerosis."

"Doctor, what big word is that?" He wrote it down on a pad, and handed it to me.

"It just means that we cannot tell for certain what caused the failure. I will make arrangements for you to be admitted to the hospital right away so you can start dialysis. There are two types of dialysis. There is the peritoneal also known as PD. This type is done at home. You can have more flexibility. You can walk with it, and do it anywhere.

The other type is called hemodialysis. This one is not flexible. You go to the hospital three times a week at the same time for a four hour session. You will be hooked up to a dialysis machine, and the nurse will dialyze you."

He talked into a machine to make notes for his secretary.

"Look Doc, I don't have time to go to the hospital three times a week.That's too restrictive."

"Okay, then you will do the PD. You will need to undergo an operation whereby a catheter will be put into your stomach from which you will do the dialysis. You will need a second operation to put a catheter for you to do hemodialysis, because you need dialysis immediately. The PD catheter will not be ready for use until a good three weeks after the insertion."

Why do I have to go through all this shit? All this bureaucracy. Goddamn, I need this transplant. Just give me the damn transplant, instead of all this waiting. Jeez, I could die waiting. I'm not ready to die.

The next day I was wheeled into the Special Procedure Room. I felt as if someone had slipped an icy finger beneath my gown and slid it down my back. "Brrrrrrhh." I shuddered.

I shifted onto a very thin operating table. A quarter of my buttocks dangled over on each side. Guard rails wedged me in place. Huge white cameras hung above. Large TV monitors were suspended from the ceiling. My ears caught the tick of the clock on the wall. My nose captured the smell of Betadine, a sure sign of impending doom. A cold chill engulfed me. In that moment, I remembered a near death experience that had occurred when I was a little girl in St. Lucia. I had gone with my aunt, Leona to do some washing near a river. As she did the laundry I sat quietly nearby. For some reason I stood up, stepped on a watery concrete slab and fell. The current swept me away and I saw the jaws of death as my head went over the cliff until Leona grabbed my leg, and pulled me to safety.

Now I closed my eyes and whispered, "This too shall pass."

While hooked up to a variety of wires, and tubes, and resembling an alien from outer space, I received no medication, no knock-out drugs and no pain killers.

"We need to access a big vein to do the dialysis." the doctor said. "I'm going to cut a hole in your neck to insert the catheter. I need you to stay very still, and keep your head to the side. Try not to move, because if you do, I will not be able to do the insertion."

Holy crap, how the hell am I supposed to stay still while he pokes a hole in my freaking neck? I ain't no superwoman.

"I will try," I said with my eyes wide open.

"Look, Miss Alexander, we cannot stay here all day to do this operation. You will have to stay still." He looked me straight in the eyes

"Well, knock me out." I stared back at him.

"No, we do not knock you out for this kind of procedure. This is a simple procedure."

"*Simple, my ass,*" I muttered as I sucked my teeth. *Lord give me the strength.* I took a deep breath, and held on for dear life.

"You will feel a bit of a discomfort for a few days."

A bit of discomfort was an understatement. This felt as if my chin was sewn to my shoulder with a tube sticking out of my neck. It would take a good three weeks before that sensation disappeared. After the procedure an attendant wheeled me to the dialysis room to begin treatment.

The sight of the patients who all looked half

dead while attached to machines made me cry inside. I knew I was entering a bleak territory. It seemed as if a swarm of bees had taken refuge in my eyeballs. A tube in my neck hooked me up to a dialysis machine. My blood flowed from my body through a tube into the machine, went through a cleaning, with excess fluid removed, and then returned to my body through another tube. This was supposed to do the work of my non-functioning kidneys. The actual process was not painful, but time did appear to grind to a slow pace. Television or reading assisted in easing the boredom. The occasional sound of a Code Blue signaled someone was in distress, creating a rush of doctors and nurses to come into the room. This caused my muscles to stiffen and freeze like a fly caught in honey as I imagined I might be next.

The following day, attendants wheeled me to the Operating Room for the surgery to insert a catheter into my abdomen. I was shocked to hear everyday conversation going on around me between the nurses and the doctors. They talked about everything under the sun. Momentarily, I forgot they were humans in a work setting, but who gives a hoot when you think you lie at death's door. When you are about to be cut open, you do not need to hear about their vacation plans, what cars they plan to buy or bought, whose spouse gave who what, what course they plan to take, what gripe they have with whom or what conference was coming up. *Shut the fuck up and concentrate on me. T*hen the anesthesia kicked in, and I blacked out.

I would come to realize that whether it was an office setting or hospital settings it did not make any difference. As long as there were a group of workers, people just could not keep their mouth shut for too long.

Three weeks later, the doctor sent me home from the hospital. The next day I felt a bit of discomfort in my stomach that the usual ginger ale could not cure. I called the PD Clinic, and was told to come in. Malcolm, Terence, and Hildreth accompanied me. I lay on a little table while Dr. Ting examined me.

"It looks like you've got an infection in the PD catheter." he said. "We need to run some tests to be certain. If that is the case, you will need to undergo two operations. One to remove the old catheter, and another to put in a new one."

"Doctor, you mean to tell me, that I get an infection, before I even get to use the catheter?"

Hildreth jumped up.

"Doctor, you mean she has to get another cafeteria."

"Hildreth, it's called a catheter not a cafeteria."

"Look at you. You in pain but you can hear for you to correct me. Nothing misses your ears."

"But you're making an ass of yourself. Telling the doctor about cafeteria, and you're saying it so loud."

"Would it kill you to hear it, and keep your backside shut?"

A sharp pain somersaulted in my belly and sealed my mouth shut.

My stomach was once again sliced, and diced. The new catheter was put on the left side. The old one was on the right side. I already had a long slash across my stomach where my gallbladder was removed. I certainly had to abandon the idea of wearing a bikini, not that I planned on wearing one anyway with my big stomach.

Four weeks later, the new catheter was ready for use. I went through a fragrance of emotions: surprise, anger, frustration, and fear. I was given a book *100 Heroes* by the nurse.

"Read this book, it will help you understand how other dialysis patients have overcome their situation."

The nurse gave detailed instructions on how I was to take care of myself. Hygiene was extremely important to do this procedure. I got a lesson in hand washing. Use antibacterial soap. Wash for a good two to three minutes. Wash fingers, nails, and scrub up to the wrist. You then rinse for another three minutes to ensure that the hands are very clean to do the dialysis at home. You hang the dialysis bag upon a pole, and hook it up to the tube in the stomach. You drain fluid out into a bag on the floor, and you put fluid in from the bag on the pole. This fluid remains in the stomach for four hours. You repeat the process every four hours.

"Nurse, how can this fluid clean my blood?"

"Think of a tea bag. It works like a tea bag to filter the blood. Now you have to understand, that you are on dialysis and the kidneys cannot regulate your minerals, so you will have to increase your potassium intake, as well as your protein. These come off in the flow. Now you are all set, and remember, extreme hygiene to prevent infection in your peritoneal lining." The nurse handed me a bag full of stuff.

After reading 100 *Heroes*, my fears subsided. Many people had more than one transplant, and they had been on dialysis for quite some time. I took comfort in that knowledge.

I applied for and received long-term sickness benefits from the Ministry. Since the Hydro blackout I had not returned to work. The insurance company insisted that I apply for disability benefit from the Canada Pension Plan so that they could deduct from their payments whatever sums I got from the CPP. I argued that was unfair, as I paid for sick premiums and CPP premiums, and therefore, I should receive disability income independent of CPP. The Insurance Company got their way.

A few weeks later the tube was removed from my neck. The PD was working fine. Life continued, and I adjusted to my new way of living.

Sometimes life throws us a lot of curve balls. We can run from them or we can catch them, and throw them back.

CHAPTER 52

ONLY THE GOOD DIE YOUNG

2005

One and a half years after I commenced dialysis I had a humongous decision to make about my work life. It was always my intention to retire at age 65. At age 54 I had to rethink that idea. Dialysis left me weak and fatigued and unable to hold a fulltime job. I was annoyed with the insurance company sending forms every two months inquiring when would I be returning to work. My workplace was in the final year of a special program that allowed early retirement, so I took that option on June 30th, 2005.

I attended a retirement party in my honour. Malcolm and Hildreth accompanied me. At first I was surprised, and then a nice feeling flooded me knowing that my co-workers still wanted to give me a send off, even if I had not been around for some time. A beautiful luncheon spread was laid out for me. I felt special and had an extra ounce of happiness when some of the judges popped in to say "Hi." I liked the four piece luggage that was given to me, as well as two bouquets of flowers.

The next day, I attended a workplace Quarter Century Club annual meeting where refreshments were served. This was a group for all employees of the Provincial government who have had more than 25 years of service. I had 27.

The following day I felt discomfort. I wondered if perhaps I had gotten food poisoning from the refreshments the day before. I vomited all day. I called the PD clinic and was told to come in right away. Antibiotics were prescribed. I was instructed on how to insert them into the dialysis solution. I got no relief, and was admitted to the Hospital. I had peritonitis, an inflammation of the peritoneum, the membrane that lines part of the abdominal walls in the stomach. The catheter in the stomach would have to be removed. A new line would have to be made in my neck for the hemodialysis treatment.

Oh God, not my neck again. My hand flew to my neck. Visions of agony circled through my head. *Lord help me. I don't want to be sliced and diced, or chopped, or cut opened, or crushed in anyway, or bruised or lacerated or scarred for life. But alas, this is the price I have to pay to remain in the land of the living.*

Wide eyed and awake, I headed into the operating room. I twitched. I twiddled. I itched. They pulled, snipped, tucked, and sent me out a zombie.

The next day, simultaneously zombied and terrified, I headed to the vampire room—aka special procedure room—to be groped, butchered and punctured in an effort to get my neck ready to help me cling to life.

Hemodialysis commenced, and the flow was not satisfactory. I needed to go to special procedure to adjust the catheter. Here I was again, in this cold room, on this icy thin table, with cold bed linens, and wires hooked up to monitor every vital sign. I was terrified, and filled with apprehension.

"Oh-oh! We cannot perform the procedure, the specialist said. "Your pulse rate is too high, we need to send you up to the Emergency."

"Doctor, it's high because I'm petrified."

"That has nothing to do with your pulse rate."

At the Emergency, Dr. Nagai attended to me.

"Try to relax," the doctor said. "I will give you an injection. You will feel like there's something heavy on your chest, but it will go away."

He injected me. *Oh Lord help me.*

With eyes bulging, I whispered. "I'm not ready to die. I have to be there for my children."

The pulse rate came down, and I relaxed. I asked for a sandwich, as I had not eaten all day. I took a few bites, and immediately threw up. The nurse advised me not to eat, as the medication would not work with a full stomach.

I returned to my room. Later, things took a turn for the worst. Fluid accumulated in my lungs, making it difficult to breathe. I was rushed to Intensive Care. A tube was put through my nose into my stomach for feeding. (A very painful and unpleasant experience) A machine attached to my nose, helped me breathe. Weak and unable to take care of myself, I reverted to being an infant, where I needed to be wiped after each poop. Adding to my embarrassment, I was assigned a male nurse and as if that was not enough, he was an Arab—known to not care too much about the females according to what I have learnt of their culture. Oh how I wished the ground would open up and swallow me. I wondered if I would make it out of there alive. The doctor reassured me that I would make it. Unknown to me he told my family to prepare for the worst. Terence flew in from Germany where he was pursuing a basketball career, and my brother Ellington flew in from Florida where he then lived.

Later, I would tell all, that I was at the Gates of Heaven, and the Lord said to me, "Get back to earth, we are not ready for you yet." I prayed like I never prayed before, and asked God to give me another chance. I was not ready to depart this earth. I still had some spring left in my waist.

Two weeks later my prayers were answered, and I was removed from Intensive

Care to Semi Intensive Care. Another two weeks, and I was back in the regular room. The line in my neck was not working properly, and I had too much excess fluid in my lungs. I needed to be dialyzed.

Dr. Nagai and a nurse walked into the room. He approached me with needles, gloves and a knife in hand.

"We'll have to make a temporary site for you to do the dialysis," he said. "Open your legs."

Open my legs! What the heck! Is he going to cut inside my jewel box? What nonsensical procedure is that? I wondered in disbelief with mouth wide open, and I could feel my eyes ready to pop out of their sockets.

"I will make an opening in your groin, and put a tube in there to do the dialysis. It needs to be removed immediately after dialysis."

I sighed, and blew hot air "Oh! For a minute Doc, you had me in crazy land."

Talk about pain. After dialysis the nurse pressed hard on the groin, and pulled the tube out. She instructed me to continue holding and pressing on the spot for another half hour so as to stop the bleeding.

I survived this ordeal.

A few weeks later Dr. Ting asked, "Do you want to go back to PD.?"

"Hell no! I will stay with the hemodialysis. I will come here three times a week, and continue my dialysis." I once again exhaled.

I had survived all the ordeals in the Intensive Care Units.

In August, I saw on TV the devastation caused by Hurricane Katrina in New Orleans, and other coastal areas of the United States. As the discussion talked about the infestation that was brewing, I was about to discover my own private storm. I soon developed diarrhea, and was informed that I had developed C.difficile, which is severe inflammation in the colonic tissues, and destruction of cells of the colon. A side effect of the massive treatment of antibiotic therapy used to get me back to the land of the living. I needed to be isolated. Rephrased, I needed to be put into lock down. I was genuinely upset because isolation meant everyone entering my room had to be masked, gowned down, equipment had to be vigorously sterilized, and the room thoroughly cleaned frequently. I felt like a leper. It is of no comfort to me being told that I will get over this one. *Am I really? They say that only the good die young and I am definitely too young to go. Still got too much naughtiness to accomplish before my final goodbye. This too shall pass.*

After having spent three months in the

hospital, I was happy to be out. I appreciated the fullness of life all around me. Feeling the sun rays on my skin brought me comfort. In the park, I enjoyed simple things like watching squirrels run up, and down the trees, rabbits hopping in and out of the bushes, birds singing to each other, the smell of fresh air, cut grass, and the sound of sun-kissed rivers, and creeks flowing. *Oh! To be back among the land of the living, smelling, and seeing an array of beautiful flowers,* as summer was in full bloom. *And definitely to taste seasoned food once again. No more tasteless hospital food.*

Dialysis came with a host of food restrictions.Chocolate was one of my forbidden foods. I, a lover of chocolate agonized about how I would handle that restriction. In the past, I looked forward to the half-price chocolates that came after every holiday.

I recalled when Terence, another chocolate lover, was little, I always bought him a solid Easter bunny chocolate. One Easter, I bought the bunny and ate the whole thing minus the tail. I planned on getting a replacement but never got around to it. As I handed him the box his face broke out into a huge smile. The wattage got zapped out of him as he opened it.

"Mom, where is the bunny?"

"It got away and I managed to catch him by

the tail."

His pleading eyes were so pathetic that all I could do was to belly laugh.

Foods high in potassium were another no-no on my list. How was I to handle this when all the West Indian fruits and vegetables were high in potassium?

High phosphorous foods, another restrictor. Nuts, my favorite. How could I resist all these? I would have to find a way to deal with all those restrictions if I wanted to remain in the land of the living. God knows I had no desire to shift into the dark world just yet.

Sparingly I would eat one of the forbidden foods. It took on a new way of enjoying such foods. I'd close my eyes as I savored every morsel and ate very slowly.

As the days turned into weeks, and weeks turned into months, and months turned into years, I regained my strength. I considered myself fortunate to be in Canada with kidney failure. Dialysis was an expensive treatment, and being in Canada, it did not cost me a thing. In addition, I had the support of a team of professionals, such as nephrologists, nurses, nutritionist and social workers.

I followed the instructions of my professionals, and gradually I accepted that dialysis was not a death sentence. I always enjoyed life, and I planned on doing just that. Oprah introduced me to the book *A New Earth* by Eckhart Tolle. I learnt many lessons from it. It helped me to come to terms with the dialysis, and to stop identifying myself as a sufferer of kidney failure. Instead, I would choose to focus on well-being. No longer would I discuss my illness in a negative light or dwell on the limitations that were upon me. I would not equate dialysis with who I was or let it define my worth or identity. I still had a lot of living to do, and damn it, I was going to keep on smiling, and laughing. A few months later my Dad called to speak to me, and Hildreth informed him that I went to a Dinner/Dance.

"What! I thought you said she was on dialysis," Dad said.

"Yes, she's on dialysis, but that does not mean she cannot go dancing," said Hildreth

My sister called for me a few days later, and was informed that I went to the Casino.

"Casino! But I thought she's on dialysis."

"What is the matter with y'all," said Hildreth "She can walk around and go places. She does the dialysis in the hospital, and then she goes home."

"Oh! She can move around?"

"Yes she is not bedridden." He giggled.

ACKNOWLEDGEMENTS

I acknowledge with love, joy and pleasure and give continual thanks to the following:

To the Great Geometrician who rules and governs our world.

To my husband, Malcolm, the poet, who keeps me smiling, and gives me strength to persevere.

To my children: Terence, who is always looking out for me. Even from a distance. Your illustrations added that extra helping hand, and love to my book; Kriston, my protector, my helper. You truly lighten my burdens.

To my grandchildren: Mya and Taitym. You add joy and amusement to my life.

To my brother, Hildreth: You have been my true champion. Always there with me on this dialysis journey, attending all kidney education forums and activities.

To my family and friends who continue to lend their ears, time, laughter, and cheer me on with my author aspirations.

To my editor, Bryan Miller, for adding clarity to my sentences. You make my writing sparkle.

To the healthcare team at Scarborough General Hospital who continues to provide me with great care and thus extend my life.

To all my writing friends at Critique Circle, Scribophile, and East End Writers Group who provided me with needed feedback.

It is with eternal gratitude I say an additional thank you to all who read my book and find something to help you enhance your living, improve your quality of life, and get to that place called happiness. It is my hope that you surround yourself with love, laughter, harmony, and peace.

◇◇◇

IMPORTANT NOTICE

Thank you for taking time to read
*A Helping Hand On Dialysis: Power Tips To
Enhance The Dialysis Life*

If you enjoyed it and you believe your friends, family, or someone would get something out of this book, please feel free to pass on the goodness. In addition, I would be eternally grateful if you posted a review on Amazon or wherever you bought this book.

Reviews, either printed or word of mouth, are an author's best friend.

Please visit Claudette at her website:

http://claudettealexander.com/

37135967R00091

Made in the USA
Middletown, DE
23 February 2019

Please visit Claudette at her website:

http://claudettealexander.com/

37135967R00091

Made in the USA
Middletown, DE
23 February 2019